6 POWERFUL EXERCISES

TO REDUCE LOWER BACK PAIN

A GUIDED FRAMEWORK
THAT WILL CHANGE YOUR LIFE FOREVER

DR. SEBASTIAN GONZALES DC, DACBSP®, CSCS

DISCLAIMER

This publication is intended to promote broad consumer understanding of the current state of various health topics as of the date of publication. The information, including but not limited to, text, graphics, images, descriptions of exercises, and other material contained in this publication are for informational purposes only. The content of this publication does not constitute advice or guarantee an outcome.

The information contained in this publication has not been evaluated by the FDA. **The information in this publication is not intended to treat or diagnose any medical conditions or symptoms. INFORMATION CONTAINED IN THIS PUBLICATION SHOULD NOT BE USED TO SELF-DIAGNOSE OR SELF-TREAT ANY HEALTH-RELATED CONDITION.**

This publication is not intended to be a substitute for professional chiropractic or medical advice, diagnosis, or treatment. Undertaking a new exercise regimen includes some risk. Always seek the advice of your physician or other qualified healthcare provider with any questions you may have regarding a medical condition or treatment and before undertaking a new health care regimen or exercise regimen.

Never disregard professional chiropractic or medical advice or treatment based on information you read in this publication. Never delay seeking professional chiropractic or medical advice or treatment based on information you read in this publication.

Reading this publication, or any part of this publication, does not establish a professional relationship with Dr. Sebastian Gonzales, Performance Place Sports Care, or any member of the Performance Place Sports Care staff. **Any chiropractic or medical decision, healthcare decision, or healthcare related decision should be made in consultation with your qualified healthcare provider.**

Reference within this publication to any specific commercial or non-commercial product, process, or service by trade name or trademark, manufacturer, or otherwise does not constitute or imply an endorsement or recommendation.

Citations to other sources are provided for your convenience. Dr. Sebastian Gonzales and Performance Place Sports Care, individually and collectively, accept no liability for any cited sources or the contents of any cited source, which may change without notice. If you choose to read or further research any source cited in this publication, you do so at your own risk.

In the event of a medical emergency, immediately contact your doctor or call 9-1-1.

TABLE OF CONTENTS

6 POWERFUL EXERCISES

TO REDUCE LOWER BACK PAIN

INTRODUCTION

Congratulations for getting this book.

Even though this book may be short, it is packed full of some of the most useful information you'll ever find on a ROADMAP for recovering from lower back pain.

Through this book, I'll be showing a framework of how to fully recover from lower back pain. Not all of the parts are included for a reason. Performing steps of recovery too soon will result in failure. Choosing and designing your roadmap is step one.

The goal of this short book is simply to give you hope, show you some easy wins. The methods included in this book have been clinically tested at my clinic, Performance Place Sports Care.

Choose to have an open mind, understand what your body is telling you and consider your next steps. It's mind blowing how quickly low back pain can be eradicated, yielding an enjoyable life.

Mind blowing!

Let's get right to it!

Enjoy!

Sebastian

USING PAIN AS YOUR ASSET

Pain is not here to punish you. Pain is here to protect you. Just like when you touch a hot pan, pain tells you when you're doing something that is not right for your body. For this reason, paying attention to your pain can be an asset as you work on recovery.

- *What makes your pain increase and decrease?*
- *In what positions do you have no pain?*
- *In what positions do you have a lot of pain?*
- *How can you use pain to find control over your situation?*

Pain truly can be an asset to your recovery if you allow it. This is why numbing pain with medication, ice and heat can slow your process because it removes your body's alarm system.

Now pay attention, because this is a game changer.

Let's get started.

"MAP A LOAD" RECOVERY FRAMEWORK

To make rehab simple, I've created the ***MAP a Load Framework***.

M – *Modify Pain*

A – *Activate The Support System*

P – *Pattern A Motion*

A Load – *Adding Load When Ready (NOT IN THIS BOOK)*

This framework will serve to answer the following questions:

- *Should I do these exercises as a warm up?*
- *What should I do when I'm done?*
- *What order should I do them?*
- *Should I do my mobility work first or after?*
- *Let's get into each part of this framework.*

M – Modify Pain

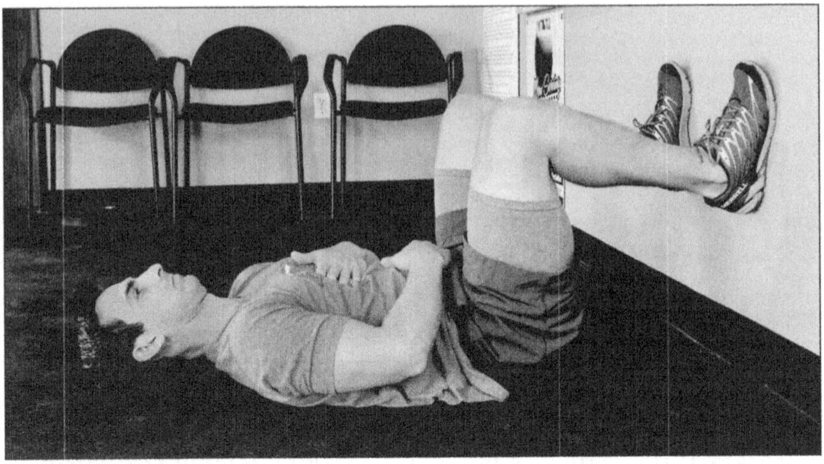

How long should this be done?

I've met people who have done everything EXCEPT the "M" (modification of pain). They do core work, stretch, massage, adjust and lift weights. Finding your body's ideal way to "cool things down" is the missing link for many people. I'll be covering a few common cool downs later.

Building spinal support systems and patterning/correcting movement patterns with exercise is always recommended, yet it is more productive AFTER we have found a natural, *drug-free* way to decrease pain.

Pain corrupts and alters movement. Modification of pain allows us to build support without the "no pain, no gain" mentality. Modification of your pain or symptoms can be accomplished in lots of different ways.

In this book, I'll show you my 3 favorite ways to "chill down" pain, using simple movements from the **M** part of your roadmap. Using these movements, a majority of people can greatly reduce their level of lower back pain within a few weeks, without the use of drugs. All of the things you may have tried in the past have merit, but what they lack is the ability to give your body a LARGE dose of relief because most of them you can't do on your own. Specific movement "medication" is my go-to.

Massage, adjustments, and mobilizations are all great, but must be applied by someone else. This very fact does not allow you to do them often enough during the 5-10 days of cooling things down. What we need is a LARGE DOSE. After we desensitize the symptoms, we need to wake everything else up.

A - Activate The Support System

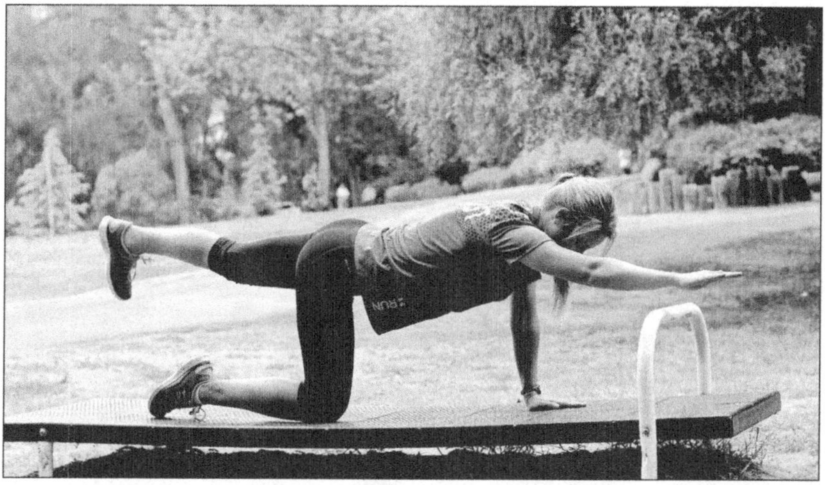

What supports the sensitized structures? The support system! Every robust skyscraper, bridge, and car has support to ensure its survival against the environment. Your body must be robust enough to ensure it doesn't hurt with twisting, lifting bags of dog food, missteps off of curbs and much more.

With lower backs, it's simplest to describe the support systems in the form of a beer keg or a can of soda pop. I personally like the beer keg example. It's filled with pressure, has firm side walls and to take it from place to place, you'll need a dolly with wheels on it. Don't worry. I'll explain more in the coming sections.

Building adequate support systems takes work. Hard work. Hard work that many people are not willing to put in, which is one reason they are having recurring episodes of lower back pain, sciatica and various tight muscles around the low back and hip region.

The methods in this book support a foundation to build from. It is by no means a stopping point. The exercises within the book will only be helpful for 30 days (performed 5 days a week), which doesn't seem like a lot, but it is.

After 30 days, the body has adapted to them and new ones need to be attempted for the progress to continue.

P - Pattern A Motion

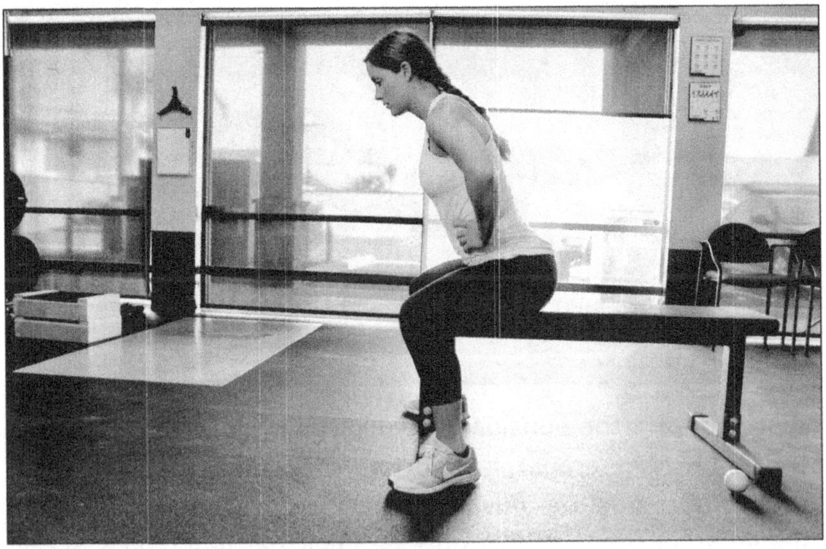

After we have decreased pain and activated the support systems, we will go through some motions that normally hurt, BUT done in a better way and WITHOUT weight. This is called patterning a movement.

If it hurts to pick up your children, then we pattern the motion of picking up a kid without the kid. If the trigger is normally walking, then we go for a short walk. If the trigger is getting out of a chair, then we may work on squatting to the chair slowly.

The cardinal rule in this phase is that we should do every repetition WITHOUT PAIN OR SYMPTOMS. Effort with a movement is fine, but pin-point pain is not.

The goal is to get more symptom-free repetitions of the movement throughout the day than painful ones. We are building a movement pathway called a motor engram.

Patterning of motion works well as a warm up prior to adding load, or even a warm up for cardio. Think of it as greasing up the old wheels.

Adding LOAD

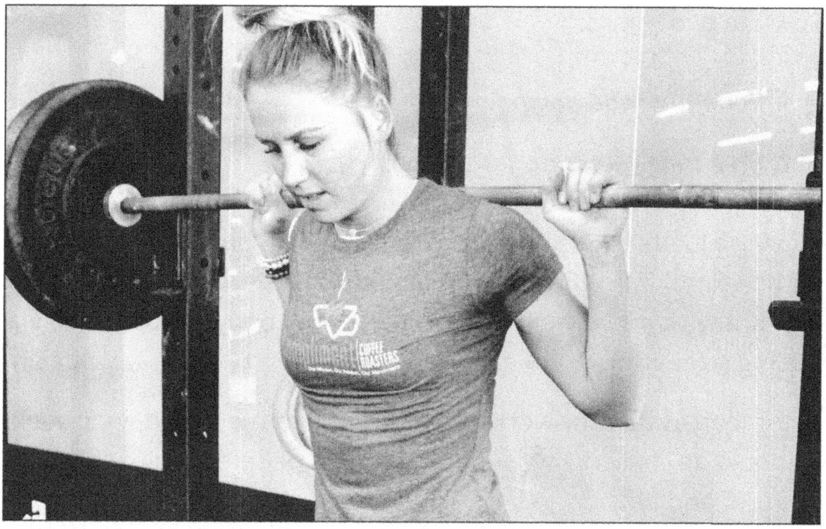

Building into load is the next step. What is a load? Great question!

In this picture, the load is the barbell on her back. Let me be clear-you do not need to workout with a barbell to eliminate back pain. In fact, many people who lift with barbells have back pain. Learning to navigate some loads that you will encounter weekly is very useful.

Do you have a dog? The bag of dog food is the load of 50 lbs. It would make sense to build enough skill and strength to safely move the bag of dog food from the car to the house.

Do you have a child? Car seats, strollers, backpack and your child all have various loads that it would make logical sense to build enough strength to move around.

If you don't have a kid or dog, you will still encounter loads. Dragging carry-on luggage through an airport creates a rotational load on the body. Getting up from the floor also requires your body to command body weight/ gravity.

Why do you think babies hate tummy time? It's a lot of time working against load!

How can you do this? Just like babies getting strong enough to walk, it doesn't happen overnight. Learning to move loads safely comes down to two things:

1. *Patterning non-painful movement*
2. *Preparing your body for the load*

Moving a load / barbell / kettlebell / dumbbell / sandbag / your own body weight through various movements / exercises is the way to learn how to move well AND prepare your body for the load, via adding strength.

Using load as therapy works well when performed 2-3 days a week. It should be challenging, but doable. Most people require coaching on form and tension.

You can do this. It's simple to do, yet not easy. It takes work and dedication on your part. Diamonds are built with pressure, and so are you. All you need is a roadmap for success.

Should you be expected to know how to create your own roadmap for success?

Certainly not. Nobody should attempt to battle lower back pain alone, but you must start with creating the framework of where you expect to go with your roadmap. It all starts with you!

Recovery from low back pain is a mental experience as much as it's a physical one. Coaching and support is key. So why do so many people continue to have lower back pain? Many of them don't have someone they can trust and afford.

They feel stuck in the middle of poor access to a roadmap and the high price of flying to get to the right doctor. This is one reason we created our online platform. Coaching, support and roadmaps shouldn't be impossible because of distance.

Not sure if you trust your healthcare provider's experience with low back pain? Fair enough. Ask them a few questions to tease out the information.

- *How long do you think my recovery will take?*
- *How many successful cases have you had with this type of issue?*
- *What would you do if you were me?*
- *Do you think I will ever get to do [insert your favorite activity] again?*

If you don't like their answer, find someone you feel more comfortable with.

PART 1:

MODIFYING PAIN

UNLOADING THE SENSITIVE TISSUES

Finding What Your Spine Likes

The very first thing we have to figure out with back pain is the **direction of preference**. The direction of preference is the direction (rounding or arching) that is MORE comfortable, meaning they don't trigger symptoms.

By finding your direction of preference, you'll figure out what your spine likes and doesn't like. Our spine is like a child who doesn't like vegetables. Continue to force green beans on to their plate and you'll be met with a battle. Give them cookies and they will smile.

This may not be the best way to feed a growing child but it works well for the spine. Do what your spine doesn't like and you will be met with pain telling you to stop. As you force your spine more into what it doesn't like, the pain will increase. Give it what it likes and it will smile just like the child.

Finding what makes your spine smile takes some time paying attention to what movements dull or spike your pain. We call this direction of preference (smiles) and direction of detriment (anger).

Many people, in their emotional state, will say that everything hurts and nothing makes their back pain better. If that's truly the case, perhaps we need a visit to the emergency room. Seriously...put the book down and get to the ER.

Spend a moment and think about what movements and positions make your spine angry.

- *Bending forward or backwards?*
- *Walking or not walking?*
- *Sitting or not sitting?*

- *Twisting or not twisting?*
- *Stretching or not stretching?*

To the surprise of many, bending backward or forward makes their back pain drop significantly while the opposite direction makes it significantly worse. Make a note of it.

Others will say that one direction is definitely worse, but the other is not symptom-free either. This is still okay, because it's a preference. Which direction would be "preferred?" The direction of preference doesn't have to be perfect yet. Make a note of it.

How can we use this information?

We can make your spine smile for a bit, which in turn cools down some of the sensitive structures in your back. Discs, nerves, joints, muscles and fascia all respond very well to this approach.

Spending 5-10 days doing what your spine likes will cool things down and dramatically improve your ability to recover.

I used this approach when I drove back from central California in the first month of having my episode of back pain at 35 years old. After about a three hour drive, the muscles of my hip flexors and lower back felt extremely tight... and I felt like bending forward would have felt great, but I knew better at that point.

Instead I pulled off the side of the road, performed 20 repetitions of a low back arching exercise called the "sloppy push up" before getting back on the road. My muscles felt lightyears better for the next hour of driving until I got home.

I won't go too deep into explaining why this approach worked for me since it would 10x the length of this book. In simple terms, it made my spine (and muscles) happy!

Here are a few ways to help "Modify Pain" or the M or the MAP A LOAD framework:

The Crappy Push Up:

The crappy push up assists with those who experience more lower back pain in the morning, putting on shoes, bending forward (with or without knees being locked), deadlifting, squatting, and twisting.

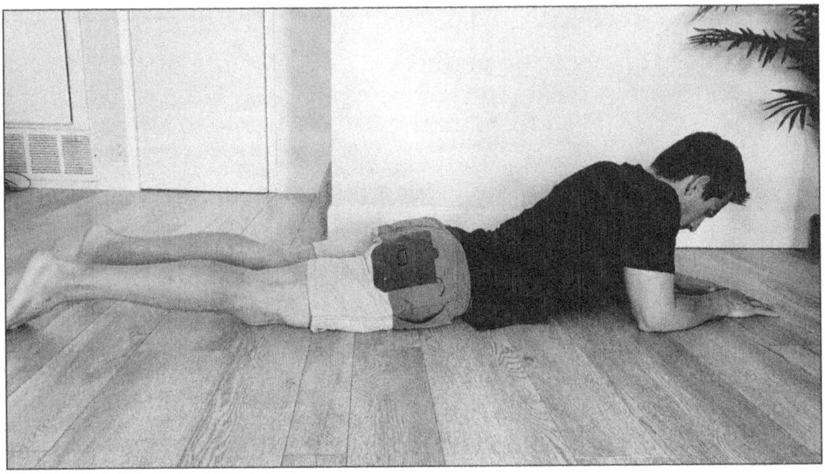

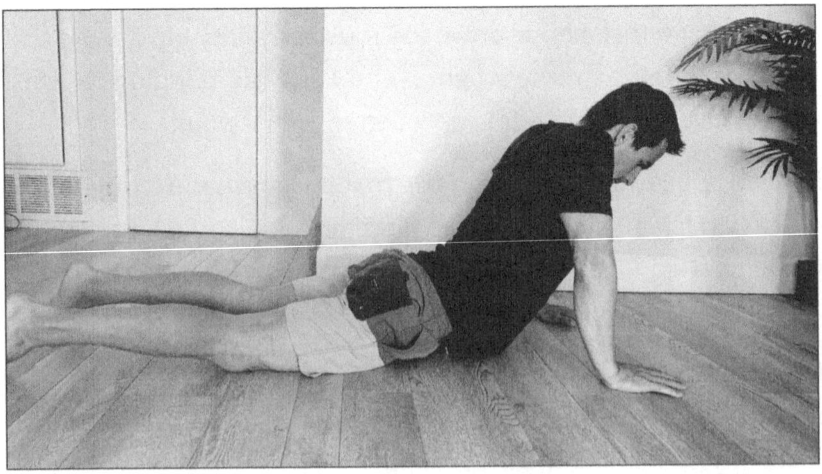

We normally have people do 20 repetitions in the morning after waking, 20 repetitions before bed, while throwing in 10 repetitions every 2 hours while they are awake. This works very well when it works. If it helps typically we have our clients spend 3-4 days doing it throughout the day. When it doesn't work, we tend to move that person to the next exercise.

90-90 Breathing:

The 90-90 Breathing exercise is for those who experience more lower back pain with twisting, having perfect posture, backward bends, walking, doing the crappy push ups, and bending over with locked knees.

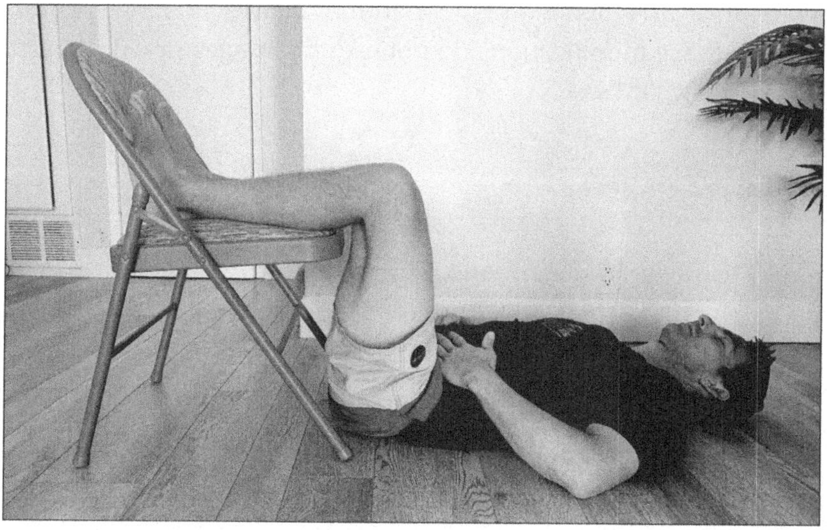

We normally have people spend a 5-10 day period where they use this often throughout the day. Normally 2 minutes, 5 times spread throughout the day is enough to make a noticable change very quickly. We also have people with really sensitive backs do this one before we even attempt the crappy push up.

How will you know which is a better fit for you?

You will feel a bit better when you're done. As mentioned before, the magic is not in doing either of these once. It requires 5-10 days of multiple times a day. The magic of the dosage effect cannot be attained when someone puts their hands on you-you can't take them home!

Modifying What Your Spine Doesn't Like

The way you perform daily activities can make your spine angry. I suggest we do them really well and modify the heck out of them since we do them often. Perfect practice makes perfect.

Below are simple suggestions for successful modification of common daily low back triggers. These suggestions will be short for a reason. You're doing it right when that activity no longer hurts. Most of these modifications do not require images or videos. Just do exactly what I say.

Prolonged Sitting

Here are a few simple options:

1. *Use a low back support and use it correctly. If you don't have one, use a pillow.*
2. *Perch off the end of the seat, allowing your hips and legs to do some work.*
3. *Widen your feet when you sit*
4. *Drink more water (it will make you stand up hourly and walk to the restroom)*

Exiting Your Bed

1. *Use your arms to push yourself up as much as possible*
2. *Don't make it a sit up or crunch exercise*
3. *Roll to get to the edge of the bed*
4. *Stiffen up your belly as you move*

Exiting Your Car

1. *Stiffen up your belly as you move*
2. *Move your legs out of the car slowly*
3. *Use your arms to assist by grabbing parts of your car*

Putting On Your Shoes

1. *Put on your shoe with your foot on a dining room chair*
2. *Untie your laces at night*
3. *Have a friend help out for a few days*

PART 2:

ACTIVATE

THE SUPPORT SYSTEM – THE KEG SYSTEM

Your lower back smiles when the rest of your body supports it. Internal support systems are what helps give your spine a chance to keep feeling good. Believe it or not, your body has all of the tools it needs to make your spine smile daily, but these tools need to be sharpened.

The lower back's direct support system is what you may know as the core, but I call this the beer keg system.

When I first began training my core, I thought how cool it was going to be to have a killer six-pack, but as I began to learn more, I found the core is actually the inside. Unlike your thigh, your core is actually a hollow tube (full of organs). Your thigh is not hollow, nor is your calf. They are full of muscle all the way to the bone. This is what makes your core so unique, when compared to other areas of your body.

In the 80's and 90's the core was called a "hoop system" because of its lack of internal muscular support. Yet, the hoop system was found to be incomplete with recent research since it does not account for other parts of the core that we are now aware of.

The beer keg is a more complete analogy for the core as it has a top, bottom, sides and internal pressure. Your belly region is the same. It has a top, bottom, sides / hoop system and internal pressure that builds up against the spine from the front and acts as a buttress system. It is EXTREMELY SUPPORTIVE, and when conditioned to do what it is intended to do will decrease lower back pain, muscle spasms, and sciatica very quickly.

What does internal pressure have to do with it? Consider a balloon animal. It keeps its shape because of internal pressure. We have the same ability to use internal pressure as a support system for our spine.

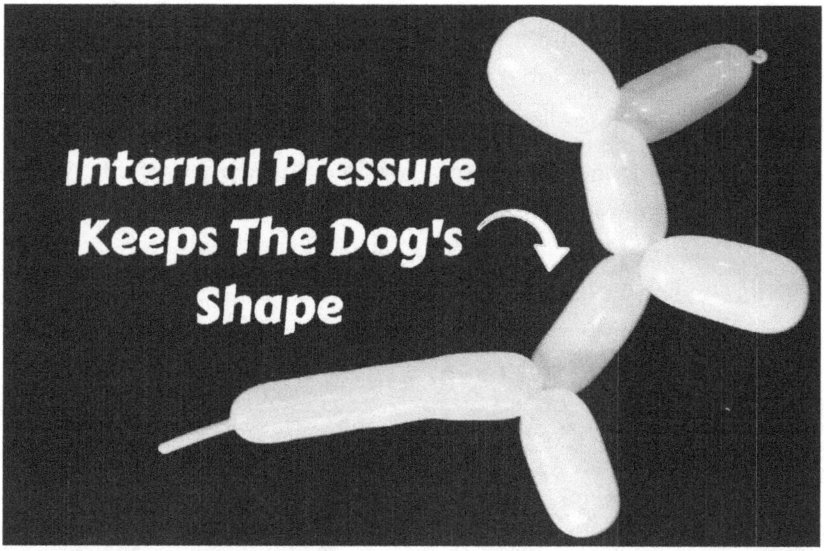

A human's internal pressure is produced by regulating pressure within the beer keg system, AKA breathing well.

I don't think it will be wise to continue down the breathing rabbit hole within the context of this book. So unless you read some of my more elaborate works, you're just going to have to trust me on this.

The major takeaway is knowing that controlled breathing is essential while doing core work. Breath deeply.

The walls of the keg system create a network of guy wires that are more for resisting than creating motion. These walls create tension to create a protective system. This system of muscular contractions assists your lower spine from moving too far from center without having proper protection.

Bending your spine forward too much may hurt, so the keg system "puts on the brakes." Same goes for all other spinal movements. Building a functional braking system helps create a resilient lower back regardless of past damage or diagnosis.

To demonstrate this concept, I'll use the following images of a system made up of a spring, wood and a rubber band. Note: the only thing missing in this analogy is if there was a balloon in the middle.

The more rubber bands we have on the "spring," the better we will be able to withstand daily life. While this analogy paints a very simple concept, it really is more complex.

I have taken some pictures of a model I show my patients about the wire frame system. Note the picture with a narrow contact point of the rubber band; the less leverage it has, the less support it gives the spring.

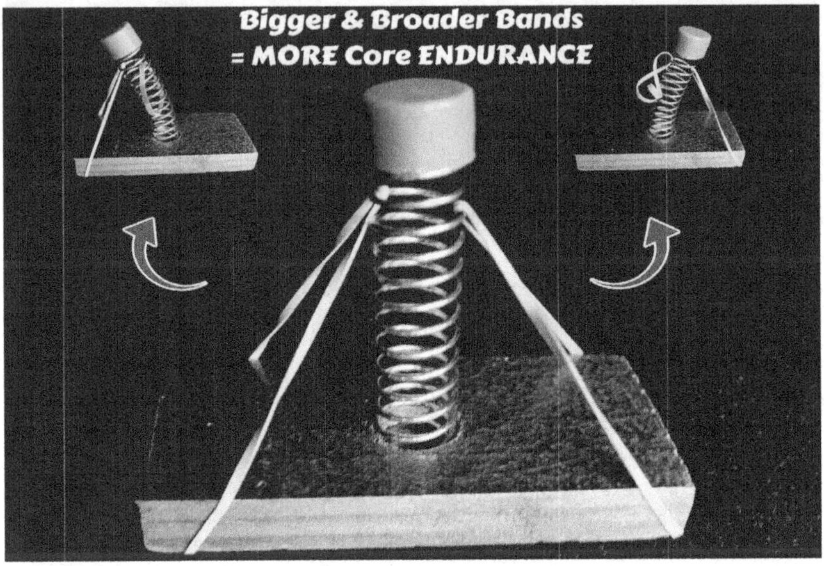

Is there more to it? Yes, but you will have to trust me.

What are the best core exercises for someone with lower back pain?

The McGill Big Three exercises (below) are the highest reward/lowest risk. However, without taking some risks you will be missing out on some rewards. Everything comes at a price.

- *The Birddog*
- *The Side Plank*
- *The Buttress Plank With Elbow Tap (My Big Three Modification)*

Note there are no sit ups or Russian twists in the recommendations!

The Birddog:

The Birddog is a great exercise for multidirectional stabilization.

When people come into my clinic, a strong majority of them get this exercise as homework. It's such a powerful exercise and when done correctly, it can greatly reduce pain and muscle tightness.

Most people are able to perform the Birddog exercise at home safely, but there are some who tend to trigger their condition with compensation movements while performing the exercise. Again, all things in life come with a risk.

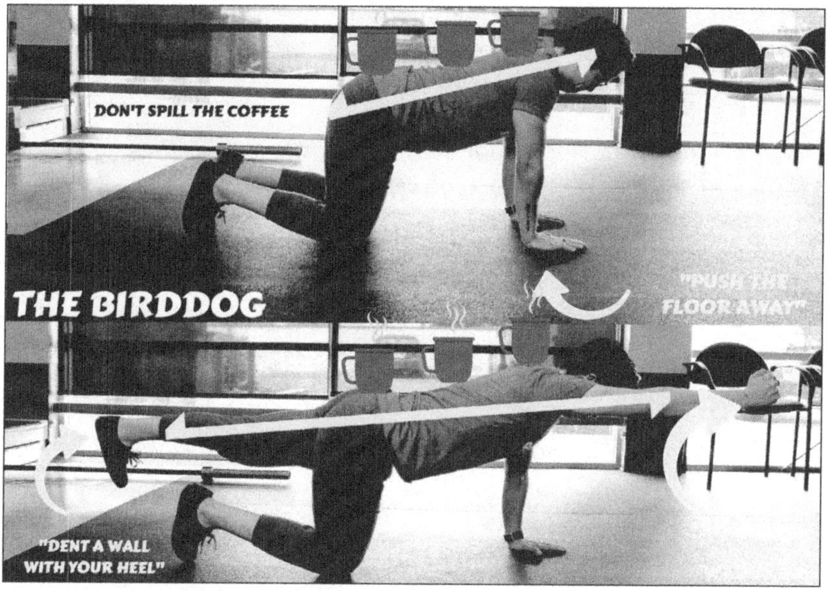

If it looks easy or you're thinking "I've done that and it's not that powerful," you probably haven't performed it with the proper tension. Tension is key in resolving lower back pain.

Here are the steps:

1. *Go on your hands and knees; shoulders and hips should be directly over your hands and knees. Become a stable coffee table (vertical legs and flat top).*

2. *Move the pelvis to find a comfortable position for the low back.*
3. *Exhale and stiffen the trunk, as if someone was going to punch you in the belly. From here on, imagine you have three full red wine glasses resting on your spine and you're on top of a white carpet. Do not spill the wine!*
4. *Pack the neck by making a double chin.*
5. *Pack the shoulder by pressing the ground away/ forcing your hand literally "through" the floor.*
6. *Start with the arms. Reach one arm out with a fist like Superman. Make an angry Hulk fist and "crack a walnut" in your hand. All parts of the low back, mid back, and neck should remain still. Imagine you have wine on your back...don't spill it!*
7. *Next, push your heels backward (opposite side as the arm that is up). Push your toe along the floor as you elongate. Finally, as you're as long as you can get, lighten the foot off the ground. (Look for changes in the spine or rotation of the hips. Your belt buckle should be facing flush to the ground at all times.)*
8. *10 second hold at the top (and always remember, you're trying to crush a walnut with your hand and put a hole in the wall behind you with your heel - this is critical to successfully creating tension), sweep the floor when you return, pause for 5 seconds and go again.*

Continue one side until you feel like you've done enough and then do the exact same thing on the other side.

Birddog Regressions:

We can make the Birddog less demanding if there's pain or inability to perform it perfectly. Instead of getting really long with the limbs, we can decrease the distance between the limbs and the ground.

The Side Plank Progression

The side plank progression from hardest to easiest is:

- *Side Plank*
- *Side Bridge*
- *Wall Side Plank Log Roll*
- *Wall Side Plank*

I like to start people with the side plank when possible, yet I always regress them if there's pain, abnormal tightness or persistent discomfort.

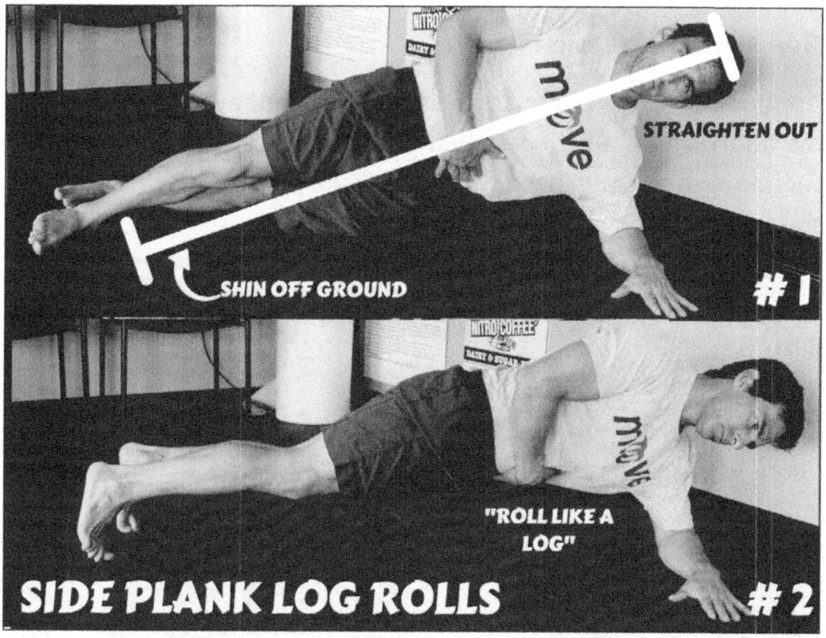

Here are the steps:

1. *Lay on your side and act like there's a sharp cactus under your armpit and keep clear of it at all times.*

2. *Positioning: Top foot in front. Elbow, forearm and hand should be in contact with the ground. Feet and forearm should be in line. Your hips will be just behind that line in the resting position.*
3. *Top hand on your belly. Breathe into the hand at all times.*
4. *Hold for 10 seconds and break for 5 seconds.Everything should be under control.*

Having issues? Here's some ways we can still challenge this portion of the torso with less possibility of complications.

By the way, there's nearly always a way to make this exercise challenging and non-symptomatic. If posture changes, or the tissue's tolerance is surpassed, then pain may follow.

Less time or less load is used to mitigate these risks.

Side Plank Regression #1:

Depending on the person's ability, we may not even start them on the floor. With many of my older clientele, I'd start them at the wall version. Leaning against a wall, in the side plank position, is a great starting point if that's all they can do.

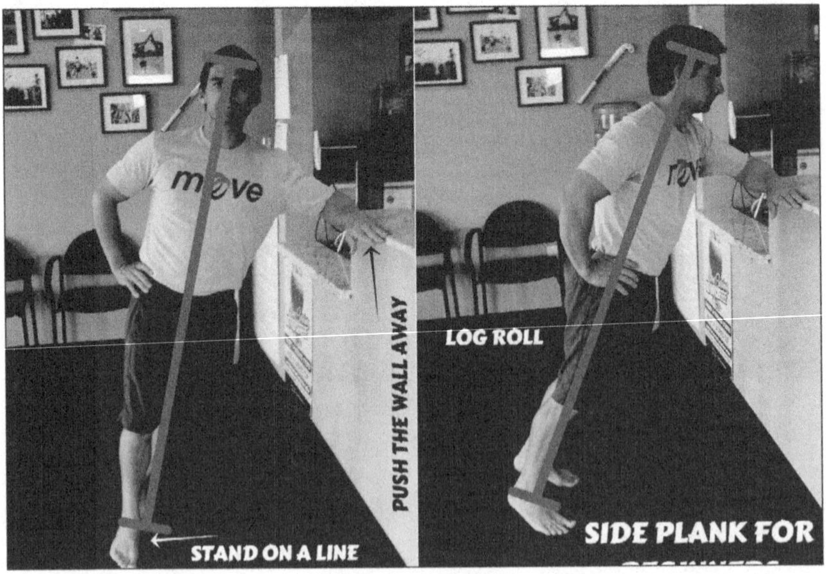

Side Plank Regression #2:

When first going onto the ground, we start from the knees. This decreases the load significantly from the side plank version.

Imagine there's a sharp cactus under your armpit-don't touch it!

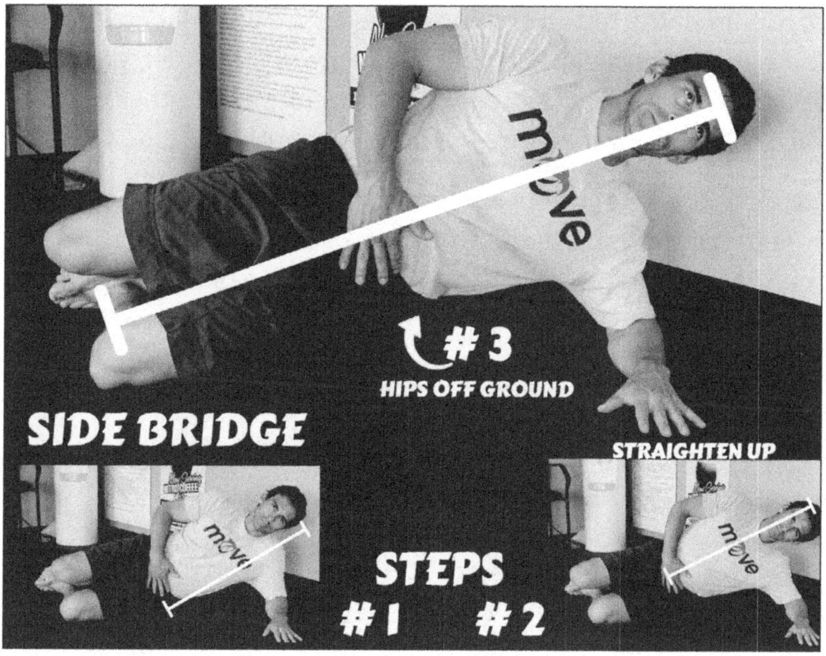

The side bridge is not a side plank. Let's get that part clear.

1. *This is the break position*
2. *Get your spine aligned*
3. *Get your hips off the ground creating a straight line from your head to your knee (look at image).*

With a side bridge, just as with the other "Big Three" from McGill, we are working on building the trunk endurance, not strength. Believe me, as an athlete you'll want endurance in this region.

Buttress Plank With Elbow Tap

The term “buttress” is a fancy way to say “remove an arm from a plank and don’t move.”

Buttressing incorporates a plank and an anti-rotation challenge all at one time. The most common mistake I see is the lack of tension through the hands (push yourself as far away from the ground that you can). Without proper tension through the hands, the spine will sag like a horse that has been ridden too much.

Here’s a picture of the proper starting point as a beginner. Make sure to not start in the poor form (low back sag) that I know you’ve seen someone do when they attempt to hold a plank for too long. This is not the way to build a booty, it’s the way to develop back pain, sciatica and hip impingement.

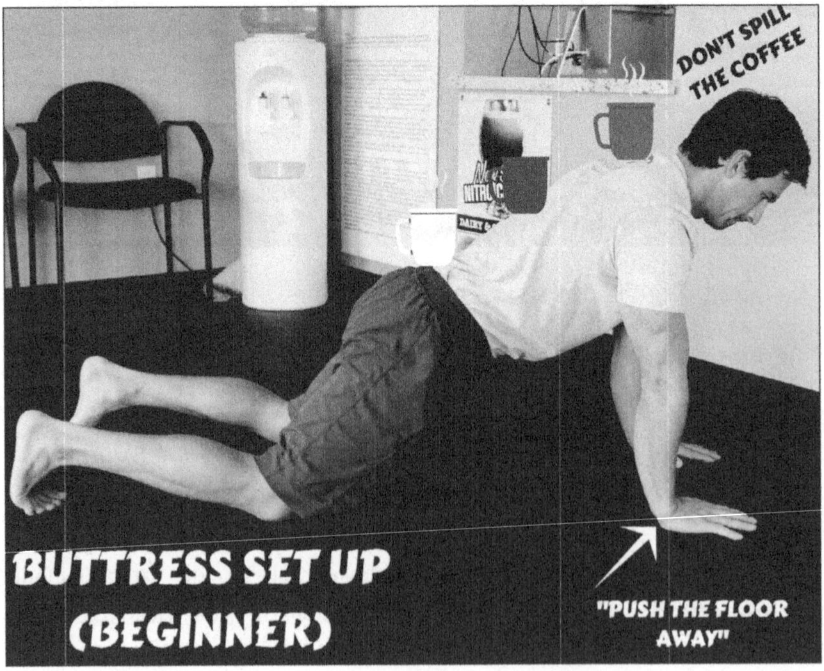

Here are the steps (some attached images will help with positioning):

1. *Start in tabletop position (hands and knees like the birddog exercise).*
2. *Walk the hands out till you find a challenging position.*
3. *Move the pelvis into a comfortable position.*
4. *You should be able to support three glasses of wine on any part of your spine, without dropping them, at any point in the exercise.*
5. *Press the entire hand through the ground or push yourself as far away from the ground that you can.*
6. *Take a breath into the belly.*
7. *Tap one hand to the opposite elbow and keep there for 5-10 seconds.*
8. *Alternate sides to tolerance.*

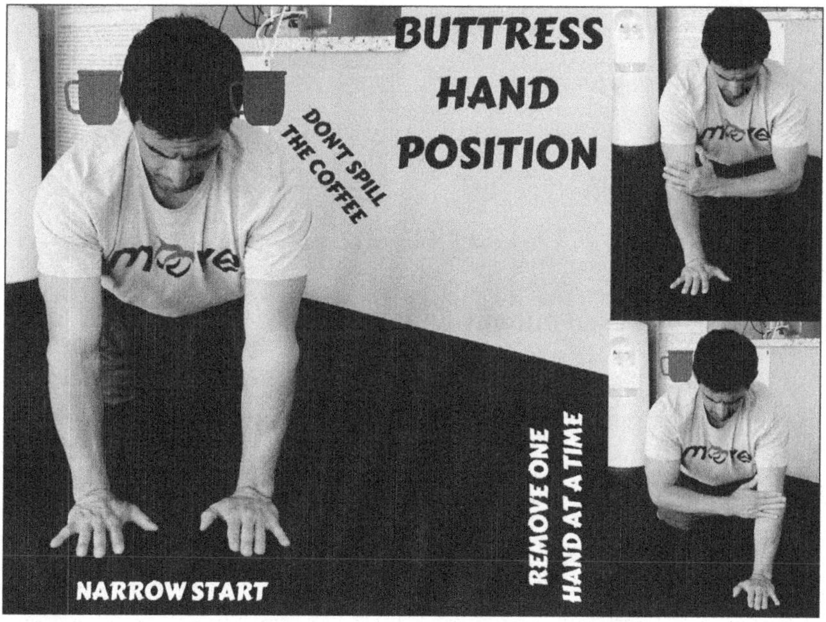

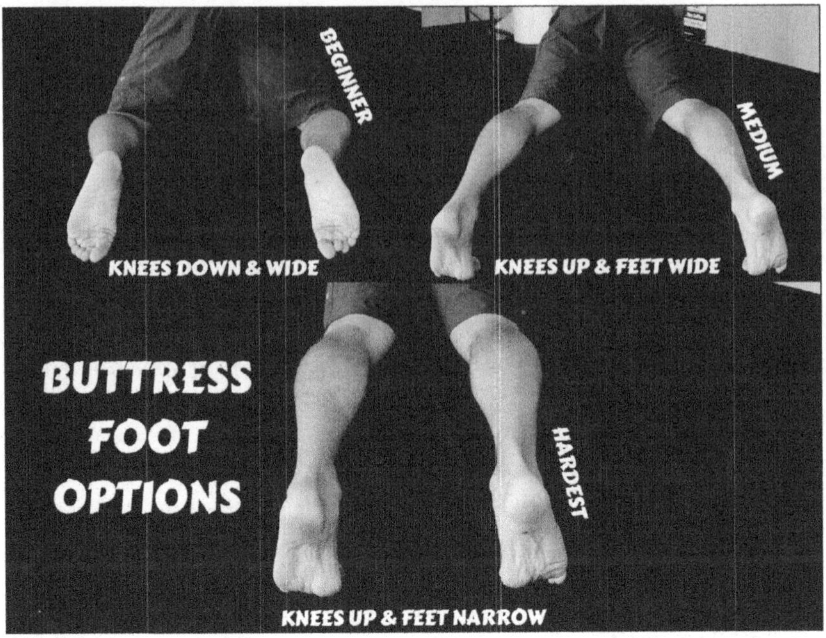

Buttress Progressions:

1. *Go from the toes if you need more challenge*
2. *Narrow your foot width*
3. *Add triple breaths as needed - Three forceful exhales "out of a tiny straw" and then "sip the air" as if it was soupy on the inhale.*

How To Use These Foundational Exercises:

Try these exercises in small doses, multiple times a day. Think of it as if you're building a bank account balance with frequent, small deposits. This will build your torso endurance just as fast as doing crushing 20 minute sessions each day, but with less risk.

Taking a 5-10 second break between repetitions is ideal to allow the muscles to get adequate oxygen for the next effort with perfect form.

For most people, I have them do this exact series for about 7-14 days, depending on their severity. Next, I progress them to different torso and hip challenges because the body requires a changing stimulus to build resilient soft tissues, resistant to injury.

PART 3:

PATTERNING MOVEMENT

When patterning movement, many therapists get very deep in the minutiae about "proper form," but using pain as our asset we can go with what feels good. One of the most common movements that needs to be addressed is bending over.

Using a dowel or broomstick, we can teach a hip dominant bending movement to spare the spine as it heals over the next few weeks. Moving with minimal spinal motion is a great way to allow the sensitive spine to heal, but not good over the long haul. Not allowing your spine to move will create other types of pain within a matter of months.

However, using this patterning exercise for the week prior to adding a load is very useful.

Here's how to do it:

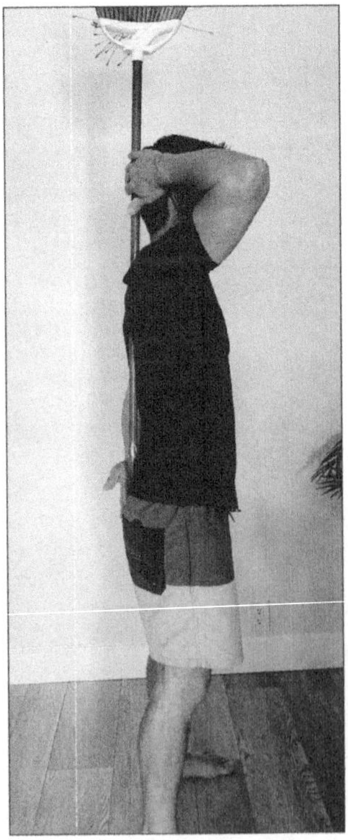

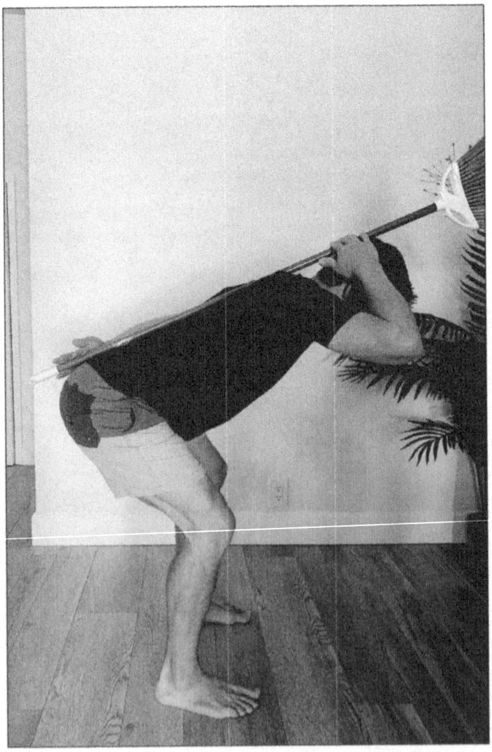

1. *Place the broomstick on the back of your skull, mid back and sacrum.*
2. *Move from your hips as you bend over as if you were picking something up.*
3. *Keep all points of contact with the broomstick that you started with.*

This is very hard for some people. Embrace the challenge. It will get easier.

This is only one movement we can pattern before loading. The squat is another biggie.

You may wonder why we are only showing this single movement. The hip hinging movement is the most important to repattern when you are recovering from lower back pain. The dowel assists in teaching you how to pick up objects from the floor while keeping your spine happy.

Repatterning of the other big movements normally comes after the second week of rehabilitation.

Note: You should not be moving like a robot, without moving your spine, forever. If you do you will end up with other types of pain.

Reinstalling spinal motion can be challenging for people and you may need to reach out for professional help to know when it is safe. A general timeline to consider is around the 5-10 day mark, yet this is unique to each person's progress.

PART 4:

ADDING
A LOAD

Load is a term coaches, trainers and movement professionals use to describe the process of adding resistance to a person's motion. Load can be from gravity, bands, manual resistance, kettlebells, barbells, bags of rice, jugs of water, changing leverage, and more.

In my observation, people who don't incorporate load into their rehab will often relapse because they have not regained hip mobility and strength to move their beer keg. They often have weak hips. To create this strength, you need to strength train. If you don't inevitably you will use your spine to move loads again, which will make it angry. Most know this as "throwing out your back."

In my clinical experience, some people are extremely resistant to doing this for a variety of reasons:

- *Cultural bias*
- *Gender bias*
- *Fear avoidance behavior*
- *They are feeling pain-free so why "risk it"*
- *Misunderstanding of loads they encounter in their lives already*
- *They are concerned they will get too muscular looking*
- *Stereotype of what load is*

Everyone is allowed to have their bias, but consider the idea I proposed earlier. Get "strong enough." Getting strong enough will not make you large and muscular nor will it require you to head to the nearest bodybuilding gym.

A common misconception is that adding load is bodybuilding or doing Crossfit. Although those are types of sporting applications of load, they are not rehabilitation of the spine. Using load as therapy does not have to hurt.

A roadmap of exercises designed specifically for what your spine likes is the best way to go about this. Bootcamps, random Youtube videos and doing bicep curls may make your spine angry, but more importantly random exercise selection is inefficient.

An efficient road map should require no more than 2 hours a week of loaded movement. A small price to pay for a spine that smiles.

CLOSING

Thank you so much for reading through and considering this framework for recovery. It works for people who have been given diagnoses like disc herniations, pinched nerves, degenerative disc disease, muscle spasms, tight hip muscles and facet syndrome for their low back pain.

We have helped countless people avoid surgery, injections and medications via this method at Performance Place Sports Care. We have become very good at helping people overcome lower back and hip pain over the years.

Once you understand how to use the MAP a Load Framework, you'll have a head start in your recovery. You'll understand what needs to get done. A checklist if you will!

Remember that **Modification Of Pain (Step 1)** can happen via many methods. From medication to massage, many things can work to reduce pain long enough to assist in Step 2 of functional recovery. It is the most frustrating step, full of questions and concerns about MRIs and talks of their correct diagnosis. Time spent in Step 1 can be as short as 5 days and as long as 14 days.

As you've seen in this book, movement is a very powerful and effective way to tackle Step 1. It is what I use with my patients. It costs less, there is no risk of addiction and they can do it at home saving them money in co-pays!

Remember that **Activating Your Supportive Systems (Step 2)**, makes flare ups less probable, unlocks hip mobility, loosens up hamstrings and hip flexors. It is needed as a stepping stone to getting to full recovery, but completion of this step does not guarantee complete functional recovery. Time spent in Step 2 can be as short as 30 days and as long as 3 months.

Remember that **Patterning Movement (Step 3)** requires practice and is a foundational requirement before building strength within the body. Time spent in Step 3 can be as short as 14 days and as long as 30 days.

Remember that building strength with **a LOAD (Step 4)** is one of the final steps in returning to a life where you'll no longer be afraid of missing a step, playing with your children, or returning to recreational sports like running and cycling. Time spent in Step 4 can be as short as 3 months to forever.

Forever? It becomes a lifestyle. Being active and loving the way your body feels amazing. It feels good to be strong and capable. It's addictive!

Ever since I experienced my second bout of back pain in my 30's, I made it my passion project to make recovery from lower back pain possible for everyone, no matter where they live. I believe the body is resilient and it wants to recover, but we all just need a user guide.

Thank you and thanks again for reading. My office is here to help if you need us. For the next steps in your recovery, visit us at www.p2sportscare.com/next-steps to learn more about "A LOAD" and beyond. We're dedicated to making you addicted to feeling good!

Dr. Sebastian Gonzales DC, DACBSP®, CSCS

www.P2SportsCare.com/next-steps

Huntington Beach, CA

LITERATURE REFERENCES

Alaranta, H., S. Luoto, M. Heliövaara, and H. Hurri. "Static Back Endurance and the Risk of Low-back Pain." Clin Biomech 10.6 (1995): 323-24. Web. 30 Dec. 2016.

Biering-SÃ¸rensen, Fin. "Physical Measurements as Risk Indicators for Low-Back Trouble Over a One-Year Period." Spine 9.2 (1984): 106-19. Web.

Brereton, Lisa C., and Stuart M. McGill. "Effects of Physical Fatigue and Cognitive Challenges on the Potential for Low Back Injury." Human Movement Science 18.6 (1999): 839-57. Web.

Callaghan, Jack P., and Stuart M. McGill. "Intervertebral Disc Herniation: Studies on a Porcine Model Exposed to Highly Repetitive Flexion/extension Motion with Compressive Force." Clinical Biomechanics 16.1 (2001): 28-37. Web.

Carey, Timothy S., et al. "A Long Way to Go." Spine, vol. 34, no. 7, 2009, pp. 718–724., doi:10.1097/brs.0b013e31819792b0.

Carvalho, Felipe L.p., et al. "Acute Effects of a Warm-Up Including Active, Passive, and Dynamic Stretching on Vertical Jump Performance." Journal of Strength and Conditioning Research, vol. 26, no. 9, 2012, pp. 2447–2452., doi:10.1519/jsc.0b013e31823f2b36.

Deyo, R.A. (1998, August) Low Back Pain. Scientific American, 49-53

Esola, Marcia A., et al. "Analysis of Lumbar Spine and Hip Motion During Forward Bending in Subjects With and Without a History of Low Back Pain." Spine, vol. 21, no. 1, 1996, pp. 71–78., doi:10.1097/00007632-199601010-00017.

Fletcher, Iain M., and Ruth Anness. "The Acute Effects Of Combined Static And Dynamic Stretch Protocols On Fifty-Meter Sprint Performance In Track-And-Field Athletes." Journal of Strength and Conditioning Research, vol. 21, no. 3, 2007, pp. 784–787., doi:10.1519/00124278-200708000-00022.

Frank, Clare, et al. "DYNAMIC NEUROMUSCULAR STABILIZATION & SPORTS REHABILITATION." International Journal of Sports Physical Therapy, vol. 8, no. 1, Feb. 2013, pp. 62–73.

Hagen, Kåre B., et al. "The Updated Cochrane Review of Bed Rest for Low Back Pain and Sciatica." Spine, vol. 30, no. 5, 2005, pp. 542–546., doi:10.1097/01.brs.0000154625.02586.95.

Hodges, Paul W., A.e. Martin Eriksson, Debra Shirley, and Simon C. Gandevia. "Intra-abdominal Pressure Increases Stiffness of the Lumbar Spine." Journal of Biomechanics 38.9 (2005): 1873-880. Web.

Https://www.facebook.com/mikereinold.pt. "Core Stability From the Inside Out." Mike Reinold. N.p., 06 Mar. 2012. Web. 30 Dec. 2016.

Kalichman, Leonid, Ling Li, David H. Kim, Ali Guermazi, Valery Berkin, Christopher J. OÊ¼donnell, Udo Hoffmann, Rob Cole, and David J. Hunter. "Facet Joint Osteoarthritis and Low Back Pain in the Community-Based Population." Spine 33.23 (2008): 2560-565. Web.

Koh, Hyung-Woo, et al. "Comparison of the Effects of Hollowing and Bracing Exercises on Cross-Sectional Areas of Abdominal Muscles in Middle-Aged Women." Journal of Physical Therapy Science, vol. 26, no. 2, 2014, pp. 295–299., doi:10.1589/jpts.26.295.

Kolar P, Sulc J, Kyncl M, Sanda J, Cakrt O, Andel R, Kumagai K, Kobesova A.

Postural function of the diaphragm in persons with and without chronic low back

pain. J Orthop Sports Phys Ther. 2012 Apr;42(4):352-62.

Kolar, Pavel, et al. "Dynamic Neuromuscular Stabilization." Recognizing and Treating Breathing Disorders, 2014, pp. 163–167., doi:10.1016/b978-0-7020-4980-4.00015-0.

Kolar P, Neuwirth J, Sanda J, Suchanek V, Svata Z, Pivec M. Analysis of diaphragm movement during tidal breathing and during its activation while breath holding using MRI synchronized with spirometry. Physiol Res 58:383-392, 2009

Kolar P, Sulc J, Kyncl M, Sanda J, Neuwirth J, Bokarius AV, Kriz J, Kobesova A. Stabilizing function of the diaphragm: dynamic MRI and synchronized spirometric assessment. J Applied Physiol Aug 2010

Kuniya et al. Prospective study of superior cluneal nerve disorder as a potential cause

of low back pain and leg symptoms. Journal of Orthopaedic Surgery and Research

(2014) 9:139.

Gonzales, Sebastian. "The New Core Training." Performance Place Sports Care, 2017, www.p2sportscare.com/new-core-training/.

Mannion, Anne F., et al. "Association Between Beliefs and Care-Seeking Behavior for Low Back Pain." Spine, vol. 38, no. 12, 2013, pp. 1016–1025., doi:10.1097/brs.0b013e31828473b5.

McCleary, M. D. and Congeni, J. A. (2007). Current concepts in the diagnosis and treatment of spondylolysis in young athletes. Current sports medicine reports. 6(1): 62-66.

McGill, Stuart. Low Back Disorders: Evidence-Based Prevention and Rehabilitation. Human Kinetics, 2016.

McGill, Stuart. "Core Stability: "Fascial Raking" to Stimulate Abdominal Wall Activation for Ultimate Performance." Http://www.dragondoor.com/pdf/331.pdf. N.p., n.d. Web. 2 Jan. 2017.

Power, Chris, John Frank, Clyde Hertzman, Gill Schierhout, and Leah Li. "Predictors of Low Back Pain Onset in a Prospective British Study." American Journal of Public Health 91.10 (2001): 1671-678. Web.

Snell, Phillip. "The Clinical Companion to Fix Your Own Back." Fix Your Own Back, 28 May 2018, www.fixyourownback.com/clinical-courses/the-clinical-companion-to-fixyourownback/.

Shacklock, Michael. Clinical Neurodynamics. Churchill Livingstone, 2016.

Snell, Phillip, and Justin Dean. "Home." Yank Away Pain, www.yankawaypain.com/.

Raastad, Joachim, et al. "The Association between Lumbar Spine Radiographic Features and Low Back Pain: A Systematic Review and Meta-Analysis." *Seminars in Arthritis and Rheumatism*, vol. 44, no. 5, 2015, pp. 571–585., doi:10.1016/j.semarthrit.2014.10.006.

Rathbone, A., et al. "Comment on: A Critical Evaluation of the Trigger Point Phenomenon." Rheumatology, vol. 54, no. 6, 2015, pp. 1126–1127., doi:10.1093/rheumatology/kev028.

Waterbury, Chad. "An Interview with Dr. Stuart McGill - Part 1." T NATION, www.t-nation.com/training/interview-with-dr-stuart-mcgill-part-1.

Videman, Tapio, et al. "Associations Between Back Pain History and Lumbar MRI Findings." Spine, vol. 28, no. 6, 2003, pp. 582–588., doi:10.1097/01.brs.0000049905.44466.73.

Made in the USA
Monee, IL
08 November 2026

68020209R00038